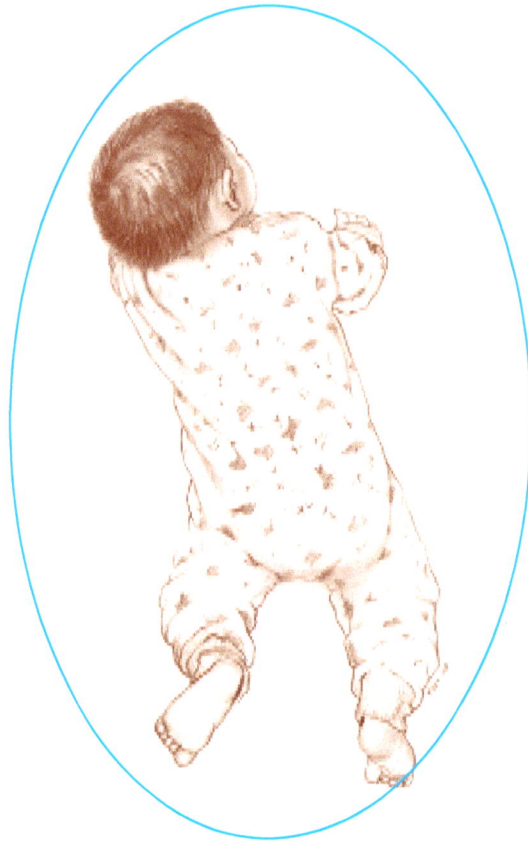

This work is dedicated to some of the folks who rescued me:

John Anderson, Marta Ballen, Kathy Young Bear, Louise Bonne, Francoise Bourzat,
James Soaring Eagle Chavez, Chief Little Joe, Ted Claus, Erik Darling, Leslie Diane
Moshé Feldenkrais, D.Sc.
Edward T. Hall, Philip Heckscher, Dottie Hill, Tay Holden,
Erik Kiers, Orlean Koehle, Bob Lefkowitz, Guy McElroy, John McKinney,
Michael Murphy, David & Linda Myers, Jinny Newberry,
Jay Scherer, ND, Lisbeth Schohl, Leonard Soforo, Gerri Thorton,
Bob and Carmen Urban, Art J. Weinberg, Ambrose Willie, and Mayer Wisotsky.

With special thanks
To all the students who continue to teach me how to be a better teacher, and especially to those who patiently
participated in the recording of this class series, and kindly modeled for the illustrations featured in this Journal.

© COPYRIGHT 1999, produced by La Escuela Feliz, Inc.   ISBN -978-0-9706751-2-5

This Journal is a companion to the cassette series of the same name and contains excerpts from:
© COPYRIGHT 1998 by Felicia Noelle Trujillo/*baby moves*™: *The Parent/Infant Guide to Full Mind/*
Body Development
© COPYRIGHT 1999 by Felicia Noelle Trujillo/*babymoves: A Quantum Leap for Humanity.*

YOUR FIRST MOVES
TO RESCUE YOUR BACK

INTRODUCTIONS

BEGINNING FLOORPLAY

BACKGROUND

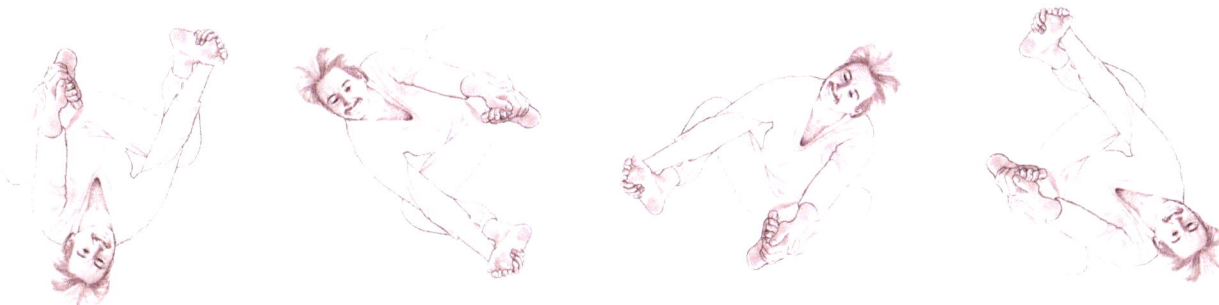

HOW TO USE *YOUR FIRST MOVES* *JOURNAL*

FOR QUICK REFERENCE
One of the most practical uses of the Journal is simply to note which moves make your back (or neck, or shoulders, or hips, or knees, or ankles) feel better. That way, you can quickly refer to each move that is particularly effective—*for you.*

FOR A QUICK TUNE-UP
There are also questions that may help you recall ideas you have had about health, pain, and what living in a body is supposed to be about. A dubious legacy of Henry Ford is that many people began to view their bodies as if they were cars: You feed your body fuel, you park it at night, and it's supposed to just run. Of course, not even cars perform without regular tune-ups. This course will guide you through the way to "tune up" your body.

TO RECORD RESULTS
Please begin by filling out the Physical History on page 26 of this book. This will help you to more effectively compare any improvements or differences you notice from retracing your **babymoves**™. You may also wish to provide your healthcare professionals with a typed copy of your detailed health history to complete their medical records, or to just keep this health history at home for your own information.

As you learn more about how we each modeled our way of moving on our parents (and they probably modeled on *their* parents), you may find it useful to pull out your old family album. Your family albums will often document how and when your postural patterns developed. Photos albums can also contain a wealth of information about your primary models—your parents and their physical postures and patterns. You may also find it very interesting to take a few photos of yourself, from the front, back, and side. Not only will that let you see your current posture, you can take new photos after you have completed this course and compare them. Just attach them to this Journal on page 7.

TO SHOW YOUR DOCTOR
I highly recommend showing your medical professionals this Journal to ascertain if any of these movements are contraindicated for you at this time. Explain that you will be guided to move slowly, gently, and only within your comfort zone—and that these illustrations are not to be "achieved" but are only a general guideline for positioning.

TO CONTRIBUTE TO RESEARCH
As you listen to the classes, you will quickly realize how interested I am in the progress of each of my students. I would be delighted to see your Journal, if you wish to send me a xerox copy. For that reason, you may wish to add extra pages to note anything that is of a private nature, so you can remove those pages easily. Each student who sends a completed Journal will receive a Certificate of Completion of this course, complete with a gold seal from La Escuela Feliz. All Journals are confidential and only used to help me research and document this process.

felicidades,

Felicia N. Trujillo

THE ZEN ART OF LEARNING WITHOUT TRYING

Let's begin by first explaining some little-known information about how your nervous system chooses to move, or not to move.

There is a famous Zen story about a successful archer who won every archery competition in the land. When asked the reason for his unwavering ability to hit the target, he gave a curious answer. "While others aim at *two* targets—the bull's eye and the winner's gold purse—I have only to focus upon a single target, the bull's eye."

This story illustrates the Zen-like manner in which your nervous system works. Like the archer, your nervous system also prefers a single, uncluttered focus—upon the *how* of engaging in any particular process. You may have experienced wonderful moments of feeling completely "in sync," when your attention was focused entirely on the sensations of the present moment, and you were amazed at how well you performed—almost without trying. When you are wholly absorbed by only that moment of dancing, or playing tennis, or making love, your nervous system can better orchestrate your moving gracefully and efffortlessly. This playful single-mindedness often generates our most dynamic successes.

Once we add a second target, for example, the *what* or achieving a particular goal, or the *who* of gaining another's approval, or the *why* of crushing our competitor (some folks even compete with themselves!), we inevitably add *effort*. That very effort tends to impair the proper neurological feedback we need to adjust our movements or to avoid injury. And so, oddly enough, being goal-oriented can actually undermine our performance.

In each case when we concentrate on the *now*, or simply focus on the sensations of exploring a process, our whole selves orient to that process. I call that totally absorbed and usually pleasurable state **resonance**, as it transforms our experience of ourselves to a sense of integrated wholeness. This state can also engender a feeling of competency and flexibility in our responses to our family and overall environment. The most recent neurological research also has proven this sense of exploration is how our brain works, how we first formed our own neural pathways, and evenhow we can grow new neurons throughout the rest of our lives.

Another Zen-like element of our nervous system is that its major work is ' non-doing!' The neurological term for 'non-doing' is **inhibition**, which refers to a blocking of nerve signals. This ability of the nervous system to stop certain signals is necessary to allow other signals to be effective. This pivotal element of inhibition gives us **choice**. Without inhibition, our bodies would be trying to do hundreds of contradictory movements at once.

Another important affect of inhibition is that ***it can release your muscles from painful spasm. This is why the rests are as important as the movements in babymoves™.***

So, allow yourself to explore the movements in this course without pushing yourself, or judging yourself. Allow yourself to simply explore the sensations of retracing these original movements, your original "body knowledge" which is far deeper than any conscious thinking. It worked the first time you created all your own abilities to move, and it will work now.

(Excerpted from **babymoves:** A Quantum Leap for Humanity, Copyright 1998.)

YOUR FIRST MOVES GUIDELINES

As a patient advocate and health educator, I feel every person has the right to information about how their body works. And, I find that even "medical" information about the brain, the nervous system, the muscles and skeleton is not beyond the understanding of any person who is curious about how to maximize and protect their own health and independence.

All of the guidelines provided in this Journal serve a single purpose—to ensure that you can rediscover your original, healthy movement patterns, learn an effective "neurological tool kit" to address a wide variety of movement problems, and reclaim your innate freedom of movement.

It is important that you wear clothing that allows you to move freely as you explore the movements in this course. The best clothing is something like a sweatsuit, with long sleeves and pants so that you can slide without friction on your skin. Avoid blue jeans as they usually limit the movement of the back, hip joints, and legs. Even spandex can restrict complete freedom of movement. Your floorplay will require a space about 4 feet by 6 feet; laying a sheet or comforter upon a carpeted floor is easiest to start with.

1. **WHEN *babymoves*™ FEEL GOOD, THEY'RE GOOD FOR YOU!**
   Whenever a movement feels particularly pleasurable, that is your body's neural language informing you that you especially need that movement. Sadly, amidst the complexities of the modern adult's life, ***babymoves*™** are one of the very few things that feel good *and* that are actually are good for you!

2. **MOVE ONLY WITHIN YOUR COMFORT ZONE.** *Do less than you can.* If a movement creates discomfort on one side (say, your right leg), experiment with using your other side (your left leg). If both sides are uncomfortable, just imagine the movement sequence—It has been proven effective to do so.

   IF A MOVEMENT HURTS OR YOU CANNOT DO IT—STOP. Skip that ***babymove*™** for now. Just continue doing the moves you enjoy and in time they will improve the moves that you now find difficult.

3. **REMEMBER, THE RESTS COUNT JUST AS MUCH AS THE MOVES.** In fact, it is the process of resting between moves that allows your nervous system to "file" the information discovered in each move.

4. **ALLOW YOURSELF THE FREEDOM TO DISCOVER YOUR VERY OWN COMFORTABLE VARIATIONS OF THE *babymoves*™** presented in this course. You can even note your variations in the *Your First Moves* Journal.

5. **EACH *babymove*™ WILL BE EFFECTIVE WHETHER YOU CAN COMPLETE IT OR NOT.** This is the direct result of ***babymoves*™** being a neurological process, rather than an exercise process.

6. **NOTE ANY CHANGES YOU FEEL AFTER EXPLORING A MOVE.** You may be surprised that your friends or family will notice changes in you that you have missed! Note any changes in your *Journal*, so that you can easily remember and repeat the moves that you found especially effective.

7. **REMEMBER, YOU CAN DO SOME OF THE *babymoves*™ IN BED.** This includes: the Side Snuzzle, Nesting Eyes, the Gaby IV, the Infant Flop (if you have a queen or king size bed and only Flop once!) You will find that the later moves are more easily done on a firm surface.

    Times to do moves include: before going to sleep, upon waking, or anytime you need to undo stress or spasm during the day.

    Professional athletes and performers also find that **babymoves**™ can be very effective to warm up, as well as to improve their overall performance.

8. **PLEASE DO NOT MAKE *babymoves*™ INTO WORK OR EXERCISE!** Not only can you get very sore from doing these movements forcefully or mechanically, but they will also lose their effectiveness.

    Remember, you already discovered (and succeeded with) these moves when you were a baby. You are now reclaiming your original organization, **not** exercising.

9. **MAINTAIN BREATHING NORMAL, GARDEN-VARIETY BREATHS.** You may find yourself so intent upon accomplishing a move that you inadvertently hold your breath, which actually makes it much harder to discover the move. If you find you are holding your breath, just re-establish normal breathing and then return to the move.

    Do not try to breathe any special way, as your nervous system knows the best ways to breathe on its own. Usually we only hold our breath when we are trying to achieve a goal. Of course, these moves are about discovery, not achievement.

10. **YOU MAY EXPERIENCE GETTING IN TOUCH WITH A VARIETY OF FEELINGS.** You may feel a new sense of calm, or experience more energy. You may occasionally feel a sense of surprise at being able to do something for the first time, or poignancy when you rediscover a long lost freedom of movement. If this happens, just rest for a few moments and allow yourself to recognize your feelings. You may also wish to record your insights on the *Journal* page for that move.

As part of the ***Your First Moves To Rescue Your Back*** Cassette Kit,
you are also invited to share your questions and any insights with me online at
felitru11@gmail.com

HOW TO USE *YOUR FIRST MOVE* RECORDINGS

And now for something entirely different! Through the window of the newest technology, researchers are astounded to discover that babies actually create their own neural pathways by their play within their environment. This means that as an infant, you playfully created all your abilities to see, to speak, to move, to rest, to love, and to unfold as an individual.

Many of us consider learning as the process of memorization we endured at school, complete with competition, tests, and proof of achievement. This is **linear learning** *and even those who succeeded in linear learning will hesitate to call it either fun or well-rounded. Humans survived for millenia without the linear learning of schools, and they coped successfully or we would not be here! In this course, you will be engaged in* **global learning**—*a total emotional, physical and mental investigation of your perceptions, your movement-- and most importantly—how you learn to learn .” (Quote from* **babymoves: A Quantum Leap for Humanity**.*)*

SO THIS IS THE OPPOSITE of every kind of learning you have done since!

1. Of course you will flip through these pages before you play the recorded classes. However, the students in the class explored all of these moves without any modeling or pictures. First, just explore the **babymoves™** following the verbal description. These illustrations are provided for you to be able to check AFTER you have explored listening to the recording to see if you are on the right track. You may find that trying to use the pictures BEFORE the class could be confusing. Remember this is an exploratory kind of learning, not the “school learning” that demands you “get it right” the first time. Do not try to compete with the pictures!

2. One of the innovations in the **Your First Moves CD Kit™** is the live recording of students briefly sharing their questions and experiences in the first segment of each class. This segment provides a wider range of information for home listeners. The taping of these shares necessitated ambient room sounds which are minimized during the actual class.

3.   As each class introduces more than one **babymove™**, you may wish to just play a part of each class and then rest. Whenever you complete a whole class, please allow yourself time to enjoy the relaxed state you are in, rather than leaping back to work or driving. I suggest taking a brief, relaxed walk after a class if possible. However, I do specifically request that my students always take a hot bath or shower after each class. Both ‘ambling’ and ‘soaking’ help integrate the changes evoked by your first exploration of a **babymove™.**

4. The extra CD labeled **Your First Moves Sequence** contains a brief review of the core movements from this course in a single flowing sequence. You may wish to note in your Journal any changes or benefits you notice from using the moves regularly. You can insert new sheets to expand your Journal.

5. This is an intensive eight week course and I recommend that you make a date with yourself once a week to do that week’s class. It is most effective if you apply the moves you learn each week at least 3 times before the next class. Please use the **Your First Moves Sequence CD** to guide you through the new core move. **Only review the movements you have learned in class.** Trying to do moves before you learn them in class can be confusing!

6. After you have completed this course, I recommend that you use the ***Your First Moves Sequence***™***Review CD*** by playing one or more ***mini-moves***™ each day until you know them all by heart. Once you have learned the movement sequence, you will find it takes much less time to explore all the moves. However, do not turn these into exercises by rushing through them, as that will not be effective. Allow your self to explore with the same quality of gentle, slow movement enjoyed in the class.

   Recent neuroscientific research discovered doing new movements ***will create new neurons!*** This is a breakthrough as neuroscientists previous believed that newborns had all the neurons they would ever possess. However, subsequent research also found that while neurons created from simply doing 'exercises' do not become permanent, **new neurons created via *exploration with a sense of curiosity* are bathed in *theta waves* and become permanent!** This is exactly the approach encouraged in ***babymoves***™—to simply explore with a relaxed curiosity. That approach is how you first created all your neural pathways, and it will work for the rest of your life.

   As you become more highly organized neurologically, the moves will take less and less time to do because you will be able to relax almost instantly. Many of my students prize their moves as an oasis of calm and renewal that they can easily access in 5, 10, 20 or 30 minutes.

7. Eventually you may find your own sequence of these moves, you may even discover new moves on your own. Through this process, it is my hope that you will own a "neurological tool kit" that will greatly improve whatever movement problems inspired you to start this course, as well as helping to address any future musculoskeletal problems you might encounter.

8. If you wish to research possible new moves that you can develop yourself—watch babies! Just do not try to keep up with infants as they are much better organized from doing ***babymoves***™ all day long! By the completion of this course, my students all gain a new and respectful appreciation of the genius of babies. I therefore recommend this Kit for all those planning to become parents--or grandparents--who wish to be "in shape" to share their baby's self-creation, as well as those parents whose backs and sleep can be improved by doing ***babymoves***™ *after* their child has arrived!

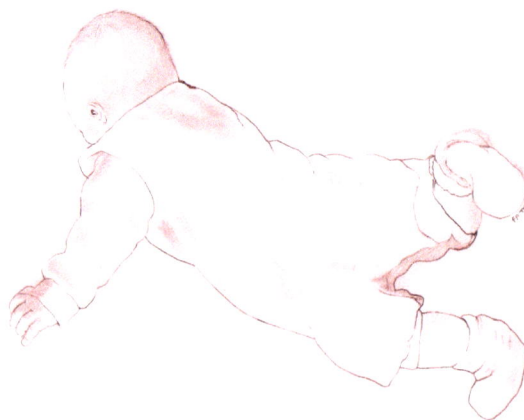

YOUR JOURNAL PHOTO GALLERY

Many of my students see immediate and wonderful changes in their posture and general carriage as they apply the moves in this course. I suggest you have someone take snapshots of you from the front and side as you begin this process, when you finish the course, and in about 6 months. This page is provided for you to affix your photographic record.

You may also find it fascinating to examine family photographs and possibly find the source of your postural habits. Some of my students simply xerox their family photos and add pages of them to this Journal.

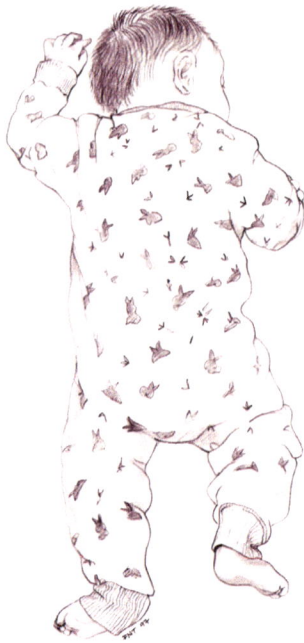

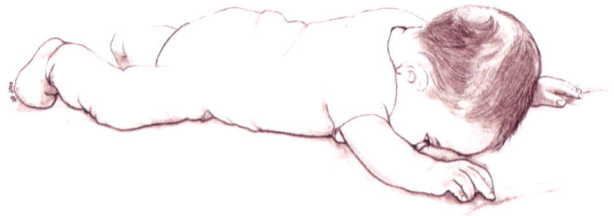

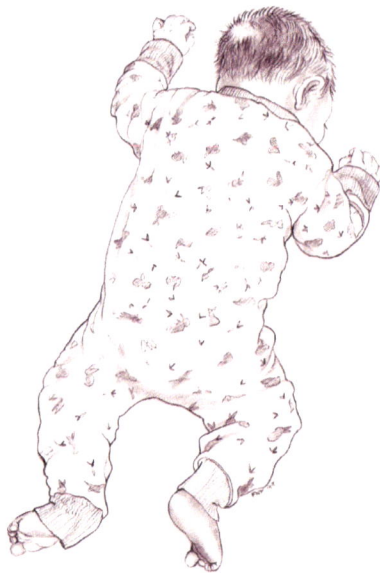

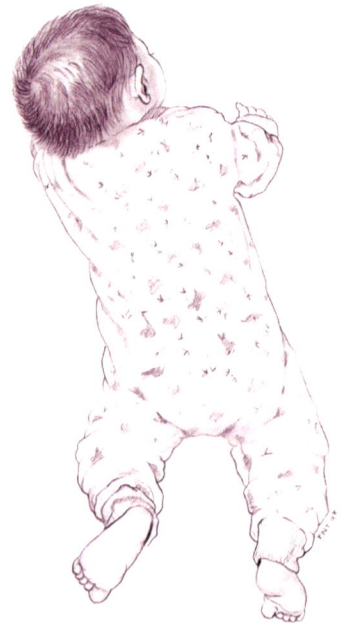

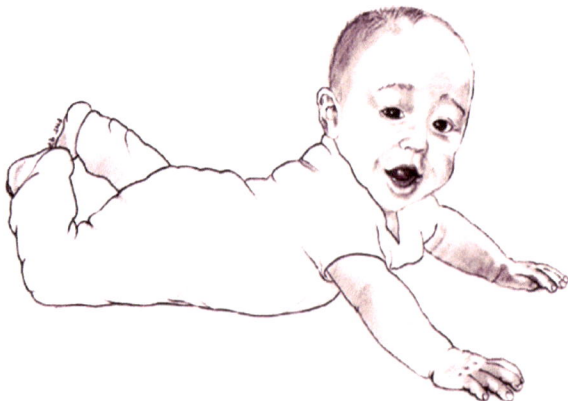

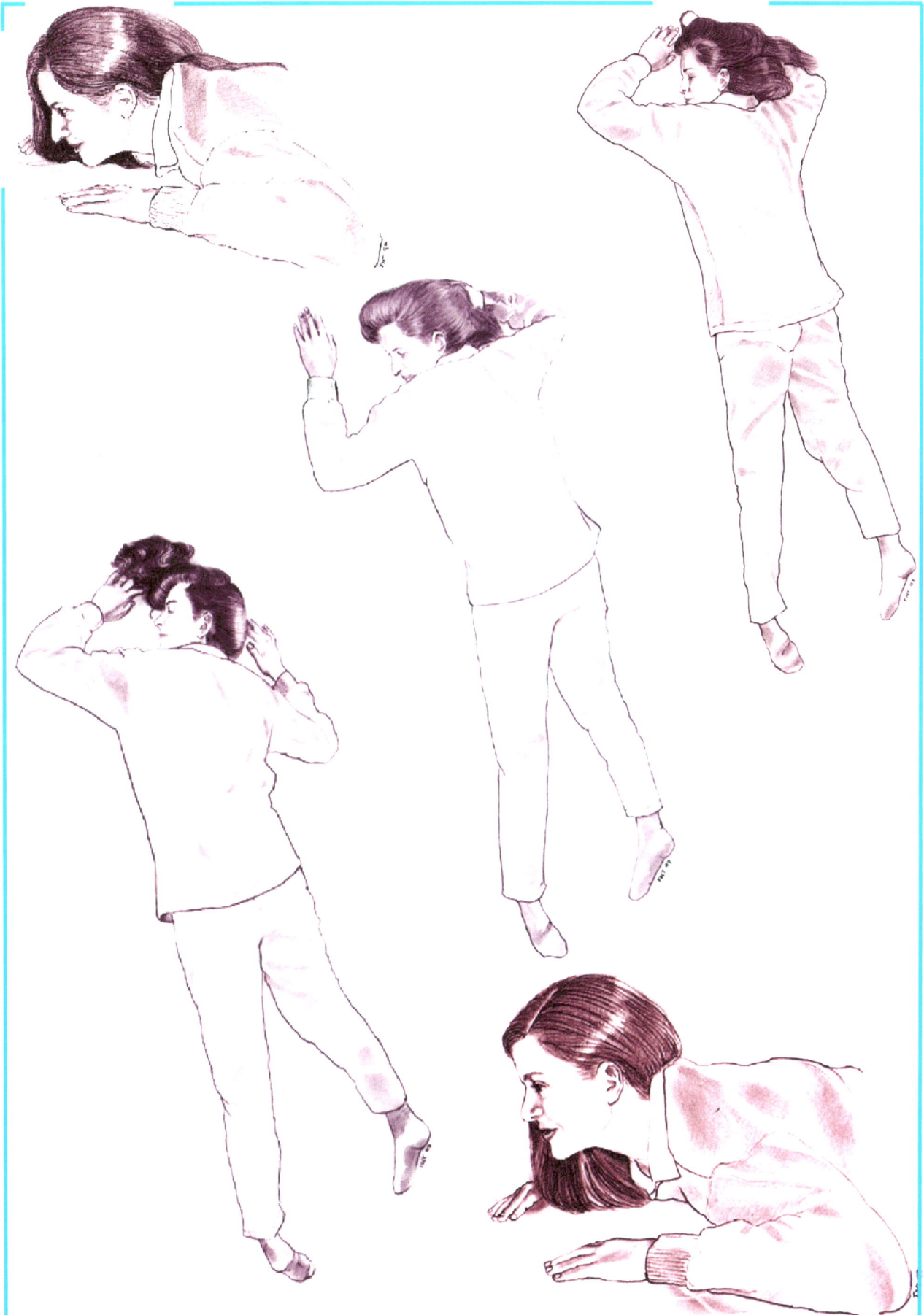

9

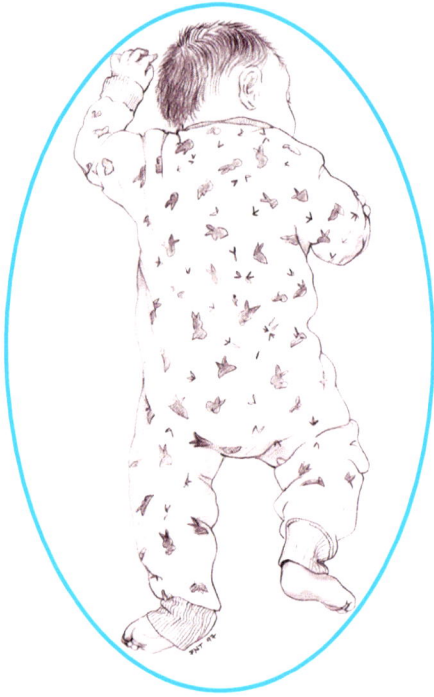

The Side Snuzzle

*One of the first movements many babies explore,
the Side Snuzzle will create their ability to lift their heads
when they are lying on their tummies.*

*The infant's seemingly random movements of
wriggling side to side
result in a neurological gestalt
that allows the baby to lift his head.*

*The baby's creation of the righting reflex results in
the formation of the cervical curve,
as well as the basis for the baby's ability
to roll over.*

*As a result of losing
this original **babymove**™,
many adults experience neck
and shoulder pain.*

*The Side Snuzzle is also essential to undo
painful back spasms
and to fully mobilize the ribs.*

*This move also recalls a sense of
calm and well-being.*

*For many years, doctors advised parents
to not allow their infants to lie on their
stomachs.*

*As a result of this,
many infants were developmentally delayed,
did not form the cervical curve, nor
were they able to roll over.*

*Doctors have now rescinded this theory
and encourage what they call "tummy time."*

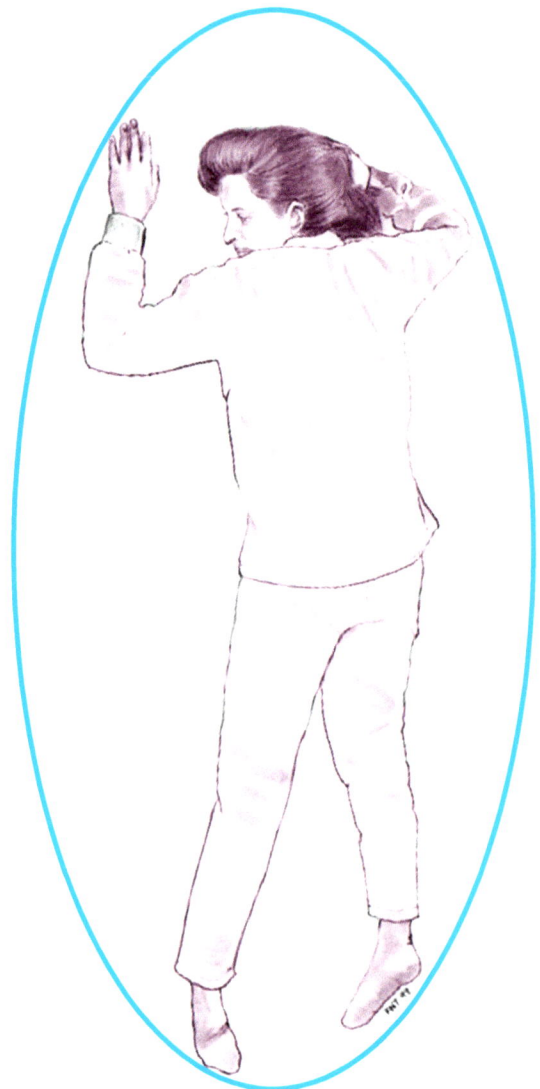

1.

SUCKLING, TOE WEAVING,
AND THE SIDE SNUZZLE

For this class you may wish to have on hand a small pillow and a blanket. Prepare to be lazy. *If you experience discomfort lying on your stomach or turning your head—* even with using a pillow beneath your chest-- please go directly to Class Three: Infant Reaching. Now and then you can check back to see when it may become comfortable for you to do the moves that require lying on your stomach and turning your head.

1. Were you embarrassed at the idea of suckling—despite its neurological explanation? Note down any feelings that arise from doing these *babymoves*™. If embarrassment still keeps you from exploring the moves, just jot down 7 things that are silly to do—and feel wonderful. If you need more space, add a page to note your experiences with using these moves over the next eight weeks.

2. Note any changes you experienced from exploring Suckling, the Side Snuzzle and/or Toe Weaving.

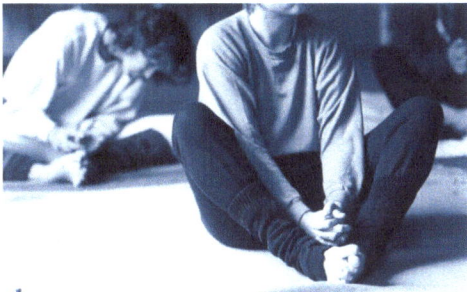

The closer your heels are to your buttocks, the flatter your back will be and the harder it is for you to roll.

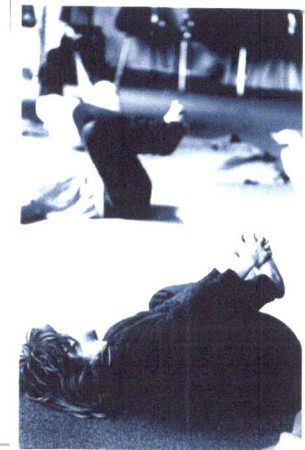

Photos by Jennifer Lovejoy

_____

_____

_____

_____

_____

_____

_____

"We must not cease from exploration and the end of all our exploring will be to arrive where we began and to know the place for the first time."
T.S. Eliot

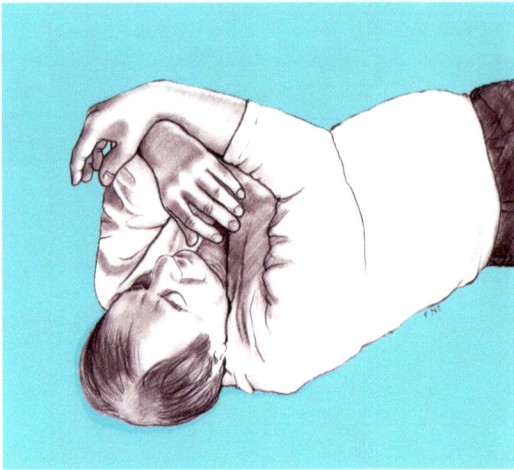

For Infant Reaching

For the beginning position--
Place your hands above your face,
crossing at about your wrists
with your fingers hanging downward.

For the final moves
of Infant Reaching

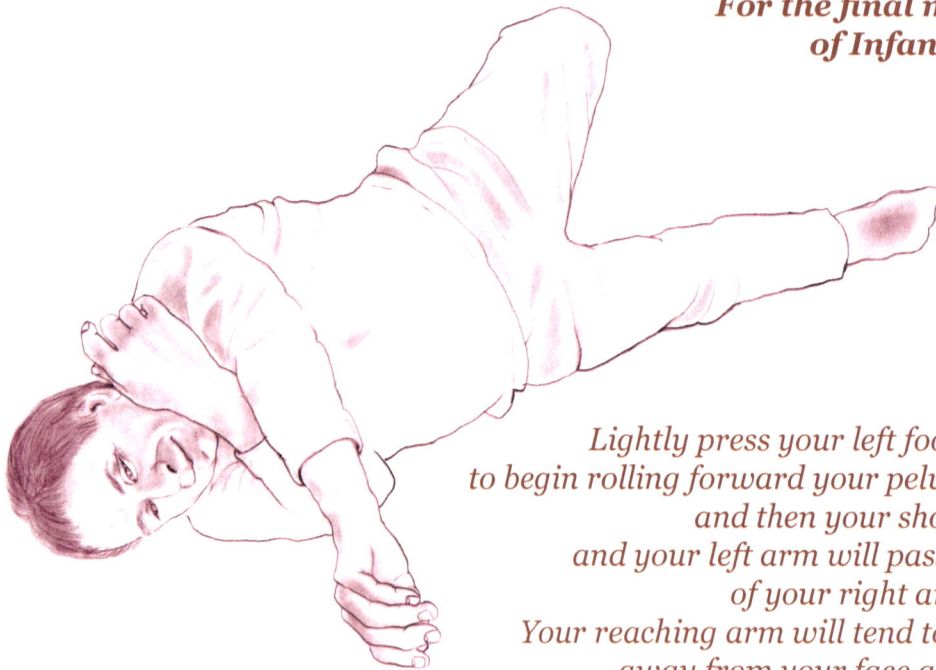

Lightly press your left foot on the floor
to begin rolling forward your pelvis, then your rib cage,
and then your shoulder
and your left arm will pass over the arch
of your right arm.
Your reaching arm will tend to rotate your palm
away from your face as you reach.

For the Self-Hug Shoulder Roll

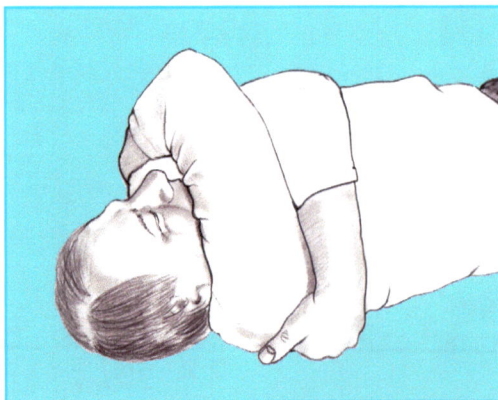

Allow your elbows to cross
one past the other,
and cup your shoulder blades,
or whatever you can reach comfortably.
Let your elbows lead,
rolling you gently from side to side.

2.　　　INFANT REACHING

If you experienced any discomfort or restricted movement during the *Side Snuzzle* or the *Gaby IV*, please explore *Infant Reaching* instead until your neck and upper body are comfortable doing those other two moves. You can check back occasionally to see if lying on your stomach has become comfortable and only then resume exploring the *Side Snuzzle* and the *Gaby IV*.

1. How does it feel to reach for something with your whole self?

2. Describe any sensations and feelings that you had while exploring this ***babymove***™.

Lateral Head Slide

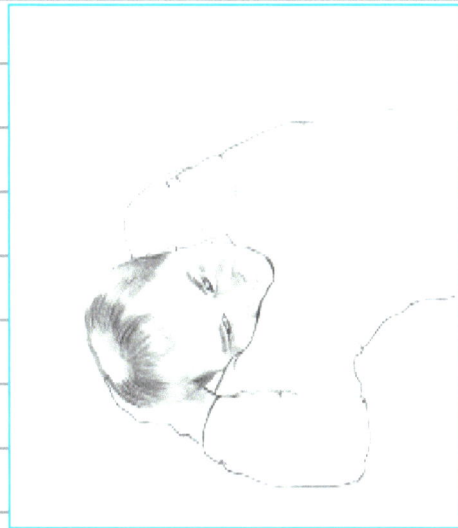

If we try eliminating the trouble without using the entire self,
we make it a problem for life."
Moshé Feldenkrais, D. Sc.

13

To begin the Gaby IV

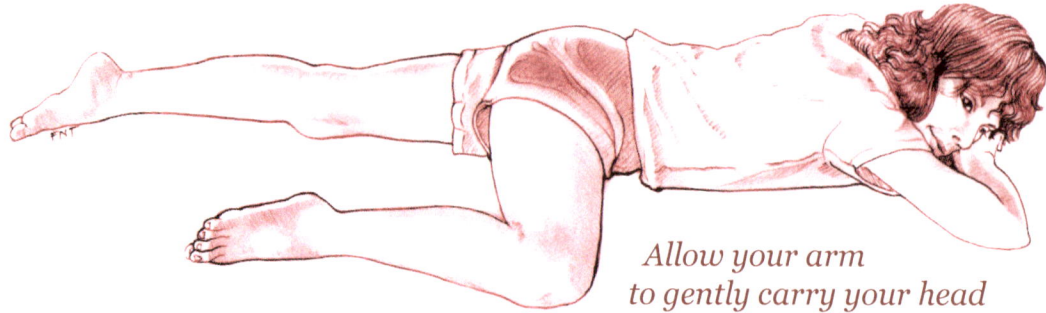

*Allow your arm
to gently carry your head
upward only as far as is light and easy.*

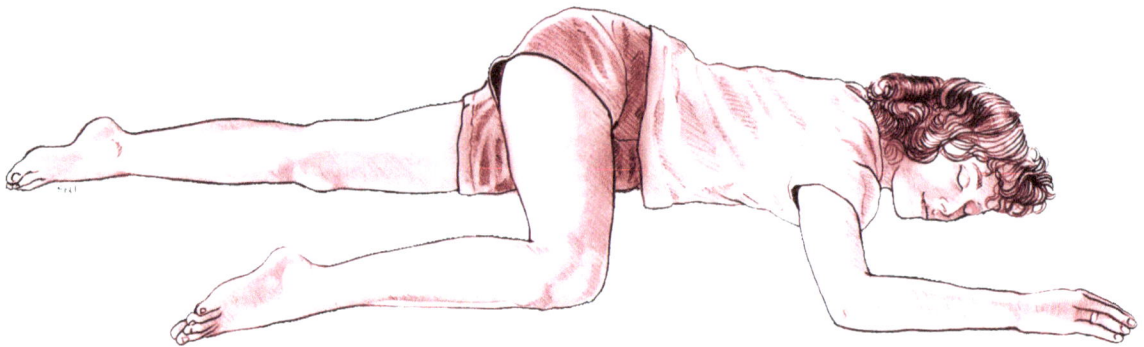

*Slide your knee in toward your pelvis, hesitate,
and allow your lower back muscles to melt. Allow your knee to slide back out again.
Rest two or three breaths.*

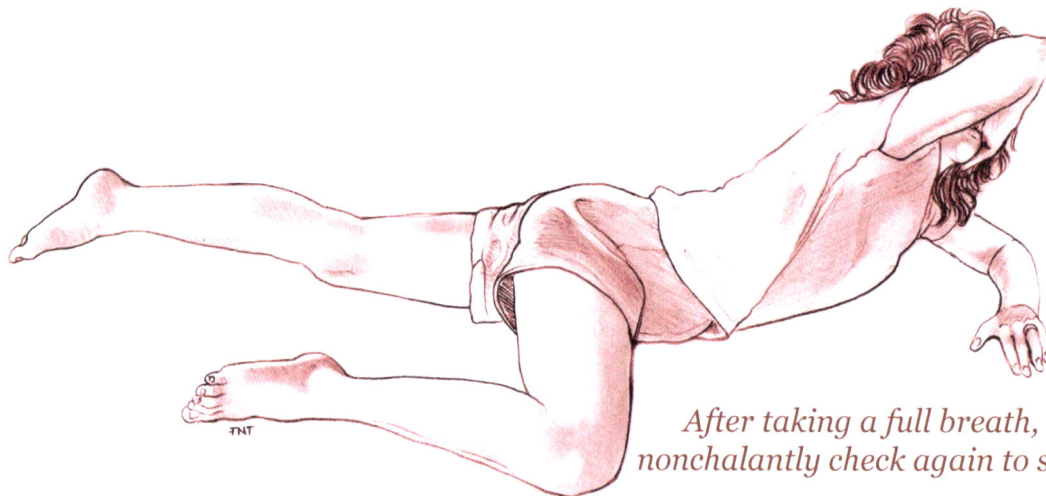

*After taking a full breath,
nonchalantly check again to see*

*how your arm may carry your head upward. Don't compete with this picture.
Linda has been doing her Gaby IV for awhile now.
Be truthful with yourself
and only go as far as is light and easy. You will improve without pushing.
Once you know how NOT to push,
gently turn your head in the opposite direction from your knee, and repeat.*

3. THE GABY IV, NESTING EYES & THE INFANT FLOP

1. As you explored the GABY IV, were you able to be a "merciful master"? For example, did you *not* force your head to turn if your neck is sore, *not* force your knee up if your hip feels tight? *If the Gaby causes your neck any discomfort, just explore Class 2: Infant Reaching to improve the organization of your neck and shoulders.*

For the Gaby IV

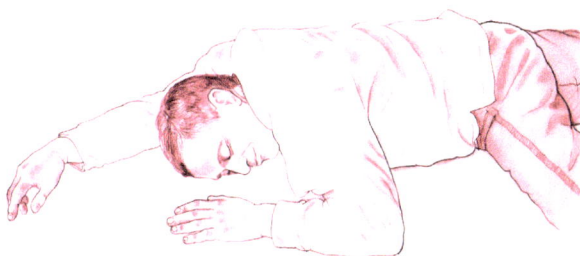

If your shoulder feels uncomfortable, lay your arm close behind your head, or along your side.

For the Infant Flop

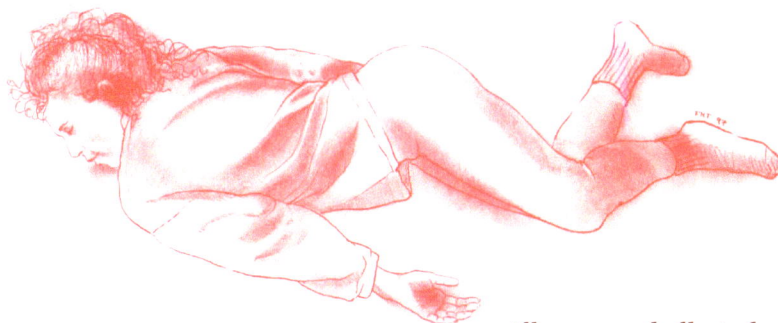

Allow your belly to lead you forward. Everything else melts.

"Faulty posture and behavior arise in a normal way in normal children if the end to be achieved is beyond the means of the child....bad postures are what they should be and would be if the life experience were to repeat itself." Moshé Feldenkrais,D.Sc., from THE POTENT SELF

15

To begin with lifting your feet

Curl your fingers and thumb
around the outside of each foot.

First, gently lift your right foot only as high
as is easy and comfortable to do.

Second, see if you can lean your left elbow
on the left leg until it feels stable and secure,
and lift your right foot again.

Third, lean your left elbow on the floor, and check
the ease of lifting your right foot.

Fourth, lie all the way upon your left side
and see if it is easier to lift your right foot now.

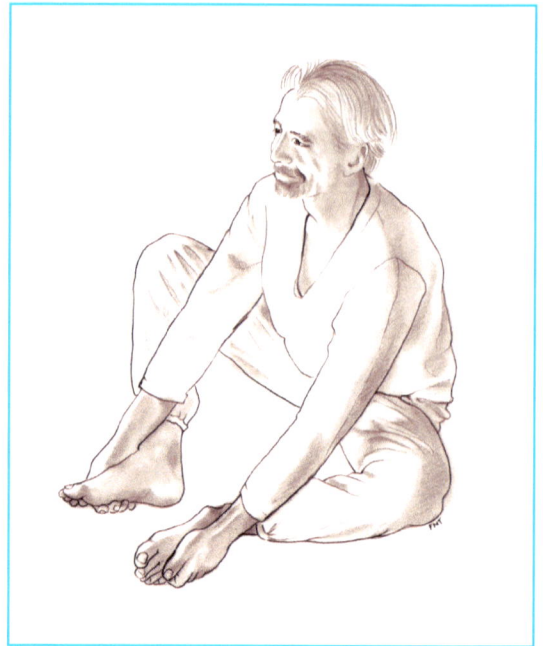

For Knee-ups

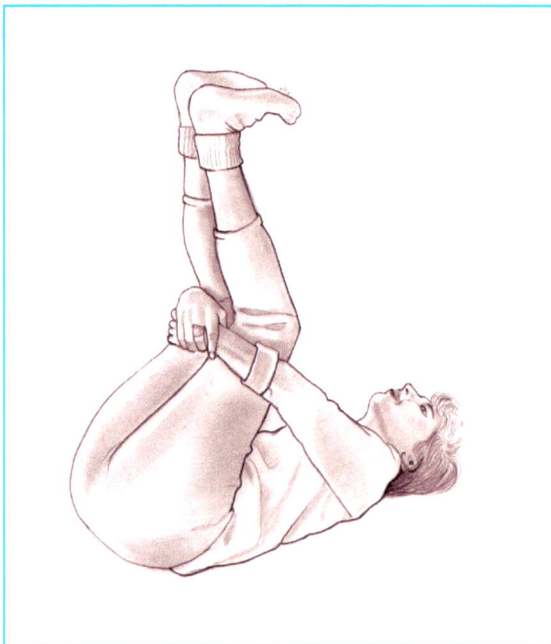

First, clasp your hands in the crook of one knee.
Lead with your heels
as if you are putting on a cowboy boot,
but do not effort or pull with your arms.

You are designed so your legs
can bring you up to sitting effortlessly.
Once you are sitting, check taking your head
toward the knee you just clasped.

Be willing to not succeed.
If you do not come up effortlessly,
sink back down and rest a moment.

If you are able to resist forcing success,
your back will improve.
And you will come up
to sitting effortlessly.
Then, do the same clasping both knees.

4. HAMSTRING BUFFET

1. How do you feel about NOT pushing, NOT stretching, NOT forcing your body to perform?

2. Did you experience that your body just might perform better by tapping into its own original "neural language" of *babymoves*™ ?

3. When asked to define genius, Moshe replied " A genius finds a way to use himself—to embrace his own weaknesses." List 3 of your perceived weaknesses and how each may have evolved to create a strength.

"What I'm after isn't flexible bodies, but flexible brains.
What I'm after is to restore each person to their human dignity."
Moshé Feldenkrais, D.Sc.

For Strolling Shoulders

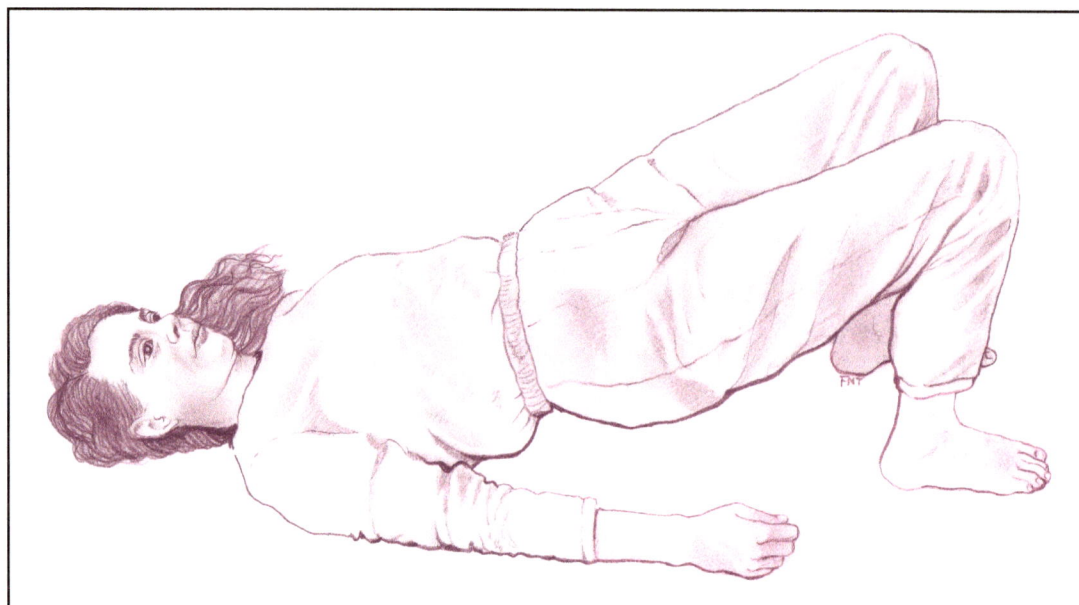

Gently tilt your pelvis to lift it upward only as far as is comfortable,
allowing your weight to travel up your spine
until it rests in the area of your shoulder blades.

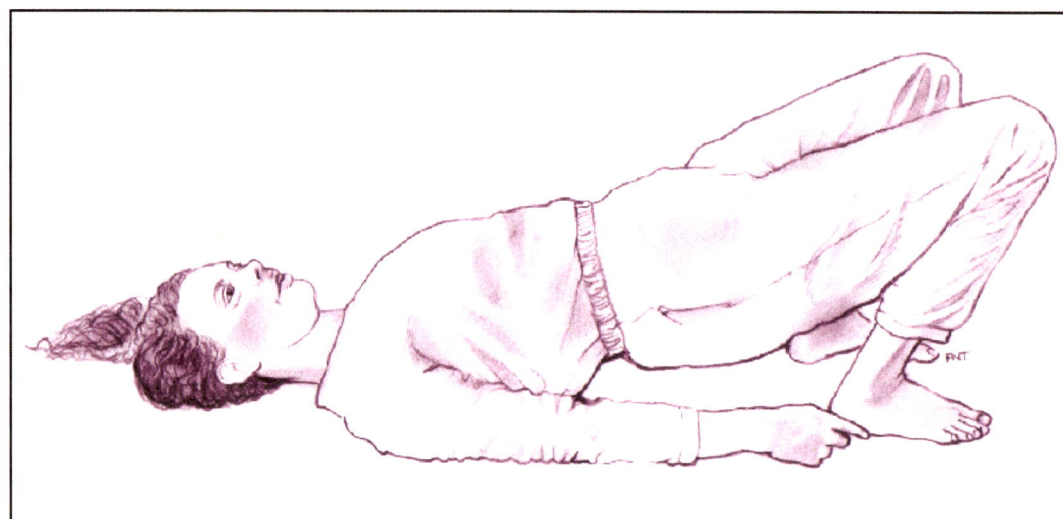

Then let your "scapular feet" walk a few steps toward your real feet,
allowing a small hollow to form in your lower back.
Then lower your pelvis to the floor and rest.
If you roll your head very slowly side to side, your neck muscles will feel different.
This will passively shorten your lower back muscles and can release spasm.

5.   STROLLING SHOULDERS

1. Were you surprised to find it is possible to walk on your shoulder blades?

2. Did passively shortening your lower back muscles give you some relief from back spasm? You may wish to add a blank sheet to record this move's effects for you.

3. Describe any "inherited" back problems or other physical problems that you feel were almost a "rite of passage" into adulthood in your family.

4. Did Felicia's story remind you of any shifts in your perception of your parents or family?

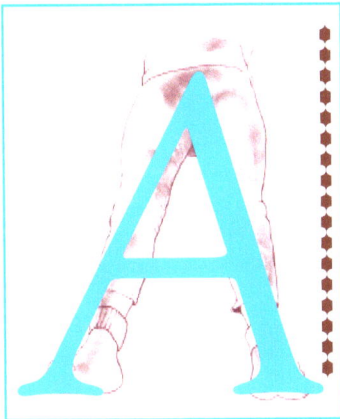

For the Leg Slide

Lie on your back, with your feet your shoulders' width apart. Let your ankle melt and sliding on the outside of your foot move your heel toward your ischium (or sitz bone) as far as it goes comfortably. Then tilt your knee up to the ceiling until your foot stands.

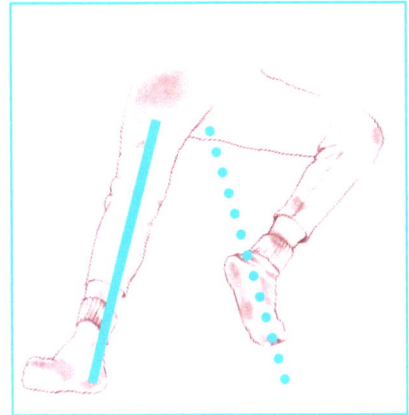

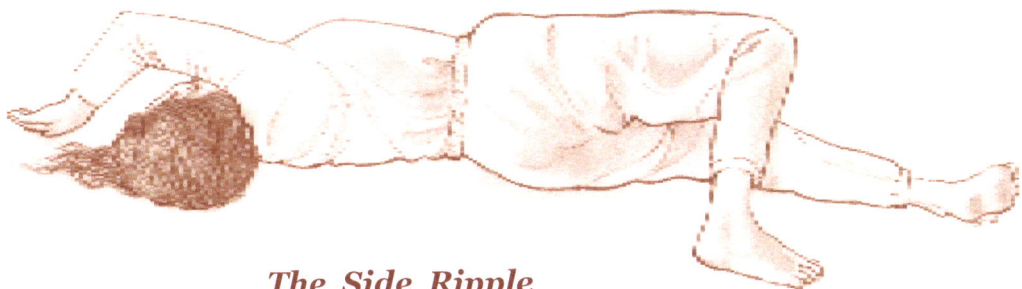

The Side Ripple

"The habits we acquire as a child, knowingly or unwittingly, prepare us for the kind of society in which the adults of the moment live."
Moshé Feldenkrais, D.Sc., THE POTENT SELF.

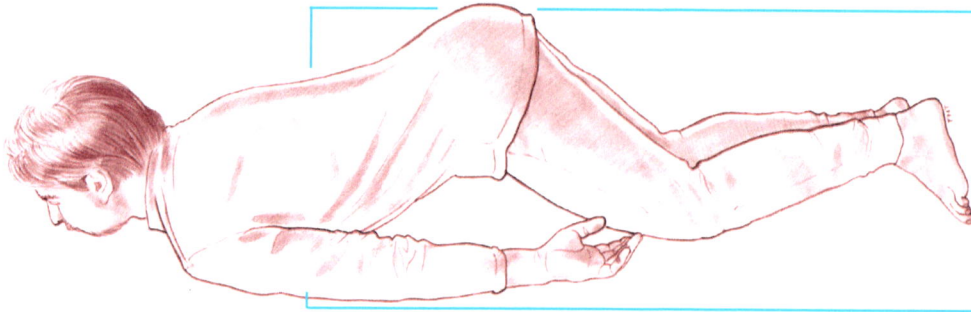

To Slither forwards

*Imagine that a soft beach ball buoys up your pelvis
by sliding your knees toward your head. In sequence, lazily raise your waist,
upper back, shoulders, and finally your head.
After each part rises, let it begin to sink so the next part can rise.
See if you can sink each part a hair forward!*

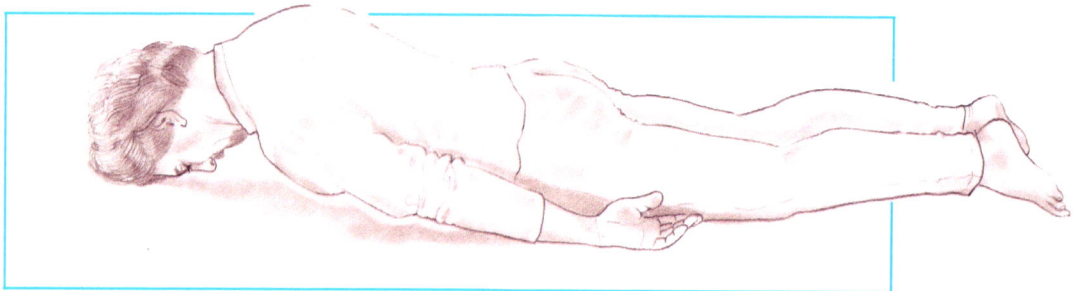

To Slither backwards

*Gently duck your head under your chest, like a turtle retracts its head into its shell.
Then hump up your shoulders, upper back, waist, and pelvis in sequence.
Your knees can then slide down toward your feet and you may move a good inch!
Or not.
Focus upon raising each part in sequence, rather than how high it can go.*

*Slide your feet toward your head.
Tilt your pelvis to create a small
arch in your lower back.*

*Then flatten the arch,
raising your middle back,
shoulders, and head in sequence.
Land each part a little more
toward your head.*

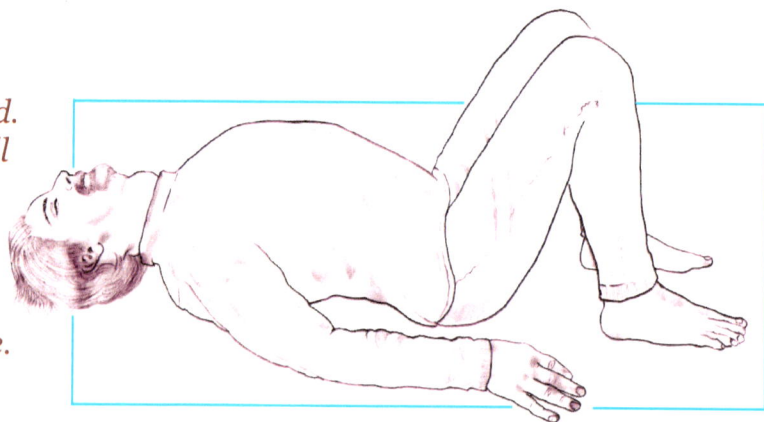

To Slither on your back

6.   THE SLITHER

1. What was your experience of beginning this unusual movement?

2. What strategies did you find yourself using when and if you found it challenging?

3. In this class a student comments, "The whole concept you've opened up for me of reorganizing and moving towards what's easy and comfortable is filtering into my life--like my work...." List any ideas that may have occurred to you about how you might make your life easier and more comfortable—especially the impractical and impossible ones.

"Effort is thinking you are not good enough."
Moshé Feldenkrais, D. Sc.

For the Zed Roll

Sit with both knees bending,
your left leg in front, and your right leg
behind.

Scoop both arms on the floor in front of
yourself
until your left rib cage rests upon your left
thigh.

Then roll softly onto your back.
See if you can roll back up to sitting
the same way you rolled down to lying.

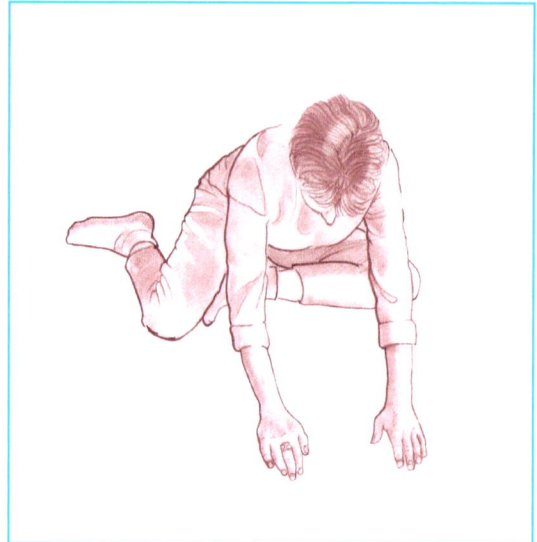

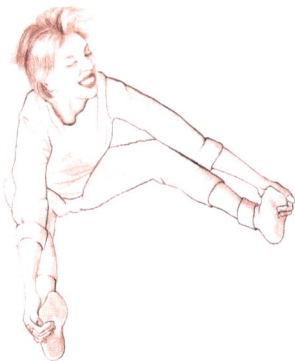

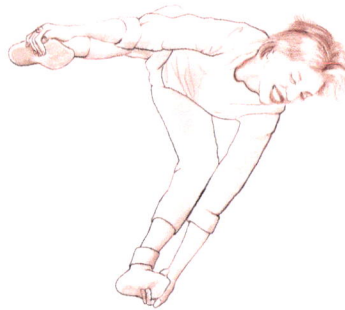

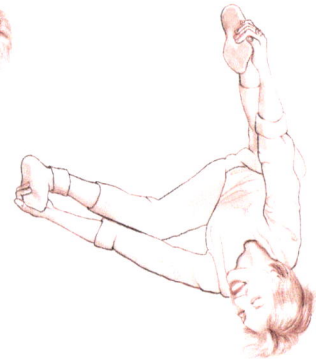

For the Bear Cub Roll

Hold each foot
with the same side hand,
your fingers and thumbs curling over the
outside of your foot.

Lean onto one leg and melt over
to lying on your back.

Then simply roll back
up to sitting
without effort.

(Refer to the cassette
for more guidance on
the rolls.)

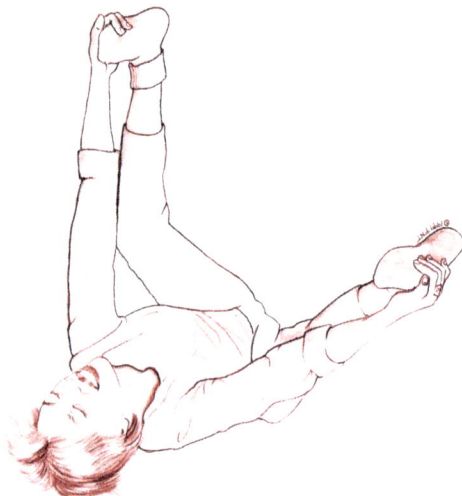

7. THE ZED ROLL, BEAR CUB ROLL, & DADDY LONGLEGS ROLL

"The impossible becomes possible, the possible becomes easy, the easy becomes elegant." Moshé Feldenkrais, D. Sc.

1. List the feelings you experienced as you explored these rolls.

2. Can you appreciate that conditions like back spasm, carpal tunnel, and neck pain are not 'psychological,' but are the result of deeply imbedded natural responses to feeling under attack? Many of these problems are simply caused by our natural *flexion reflex,* which is elicited when we are sad or afraid. (More at *www.BackRescue.com*.)

3. On the next page create two columns. In Column I, list the stressors in your life. In Column II, list any symptoms you are currently experiencing. See how many ways you

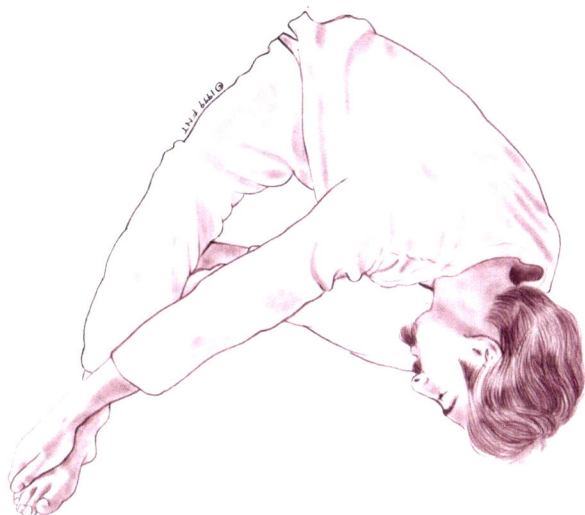

*At first,
to come back UP to sitting
with the **Bear Cub Roll,**
just extend your top leg as you roll
to one side.*

_____

_____

_____

_____

_____

*Once you have recalled this move
rolling down and up
are pretty much the same--
relaxed, effortless and unexpectedly
gleeful....*

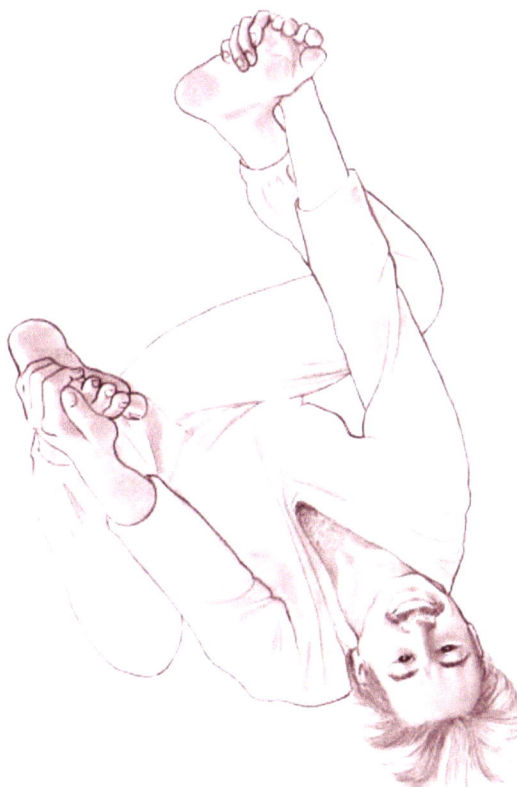

STRESSORS & SYMPTOMS

"If you know what you do,
you can do what you want." Moshé Feldenkrais, D.Sc.

8. THE MYSTERY FINAL CLASS

In all my years of teaching this course, I have always enjoined the graduating students to keep secret the moves explored in this last class. In keeping with this tradition, there are no illustrations of this move—but it is a wonderful climax to all of your training before this class. *If you decide NOT to do this class at this time, you may still address the questions for this class.* You may need to add more paper to describe your experiences fully.

You will need the following for this class:
1) To remove your socks and (if you wear them) to put aside your eye glasses.
2) To place near your mat some non-greasy body or hand lotion.
3) If your Kit is made up of CDs, completely empty your binder of all CDs and materials and then to tape it shut with short pieces of tape on the three sides that open, so the binder will not open.
   If your Kit is made up of tape cassettes, remove all the pages and tapes, use short pieces of tape on the three sides that open, so the box will not open.
4) Whenever Felicia says "**board**" apply her instructions to your **binder** or your **box.**
5) This last class has a new format of students shares *after* the class, so keep on listening after the musical interlude.

THIS CLASS IS *NOT* RECOMMENDED FOR THOSE WITH HIP REPLACEMENT SURGERY OR SEVERE LIMITATION OF HIP MOVEMENT. PLEASE ASK YOUR DOCTOR AND FOLLOW MEDICAL GUIDELINES.

1. What strategies have you used during this course when a movement seemed impossible for you to find?

2. Please list any new learning strategies you discovered during this course.

3. Please list any improvements or benefits you experienced from this course.

_____

_____

_____

_____

_____

_____

"My true goal is that you will live out your unavowed dreams."
Moshe Feldenkrais, D.Sc.

YOUR COMPLETE PHYSICAL HISTORY

I begin with each private student by taking a year by year history of how someone has lived in his or her body. An unusual aspect of my histories is that in addition to recording physical traumas, I give equal weight to any and all emotional stressors, for example: stress surrounding your birth, parental divorce, being teased at school, being taller or shorter than others, having an unusually critical parent, working for a difficult boss, difficulty with relationships, training in ballet or athletics, as well as writing Masters or Doctoral theses—as often these situations result in a stoical accommodation to prolonged stress.

As you will learn, all of these stressors contribute to a posture of "flexion"*, our genetically engineered response to attack on any level. How you have lived in your body is a map of how you were able to address the stressors and demands of your life and social environment. Please note all physical and emotional traumas beginning with any stories you know about your mother's pregnancy and your birth in the left-hand columns. Later, as you complete this course, note any insights or changes in the right-hand columns.

It is also important that you list how you felt, not just the medical terms ascribed to your symptoms. My clients have found this a very useful process, which is why I highly recommend beginning with creating this detailed history for your own information and records.

My Physical History	Insights and Changes

*For more information about "flexion" see **BackRescue.com** under page titled:
Your Back's Anatomy (What Dr. Sarno doesn't tell you!)

My Physical History	Insights and Changes

GLOSSARY

Cervical—Pertains to the neck, i.e. the upper seven vertebrae that make up the neck.

Differentiated—As applied to movement, the ability to move parts of the body separately, for example moving the head but not the shoulders, or the ribs but not the pelvis. Differentiation can indicate neurological maturation; children will often move their jaws as they use scissors for the first time, as unconsciously they have not yet differentiated their teeth from the "teeth" of the scissors.

Homunculus—(See page 29) A graphic representation of the ratio of nerves from the different parts of the body to the sensory and motor (feeling and doing) parts of the brain.

Litmus paper—A litmus-treated paper used to indicate the acidity or alkalinity of solutions. In this course the term is loosely used to indicate a measurement before and after a movement to note its effects.

Mudra—An East Indian hand movement which is used in traditional dance. In this course the term is used to indicate involuntary hand movements elicited by a lack of differentiation.

Palpate—The act of feeling lightly with the fingers to note delicate variations of tissue texture beneath the skin. This simple action can also help fill in the internal image and by giving this simple input, the brain can react by reorganizing the area palpated.

Resonance—The sensation of feeling completely "in sync" or wholly absorbed by exploring a process rather than efforting to achieve a goal, to compete, or to gain another's approval. I have named that totally focused and usually pleasurable state **resonance**, as this state can also engender a feeling of competency and flexibility in our overall environment.

Scapulae—The two shoulder blades which are flat triangular bones located on the upper back and work as part of the shoulder articulations. The full movement of the scapulae would include sliding in a circular motion, as well as moving toward and away from the spine, and upward or downward relative to the head and feet. See Illustrations on page 29.

Somatic koan—Originally 'koan' is a Zen riddle and 'somatic' is a term describing the experience of one's own body. I coined this phrase to describe a method of teaching that presents koans, or riddles, to invite exploration of one's somatic experience.

Trajectory—The path that a body or parts of a body inscribe in space. For example, this is used to describe the path a foot or arm takes from one position to another.

Witness—Is used in this course to denote a relaxed, playful observation of oneself without acting to "improve" or change one's actions. For example, while doing a **babymove**™ the

KNOWING WHAT YOU ARE MOVING

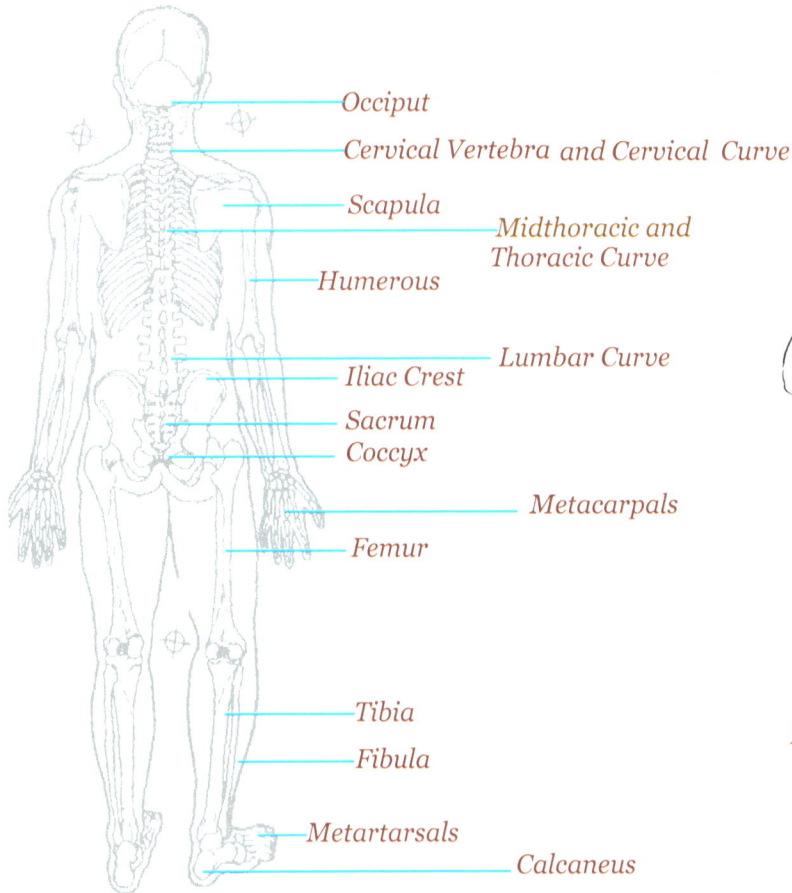

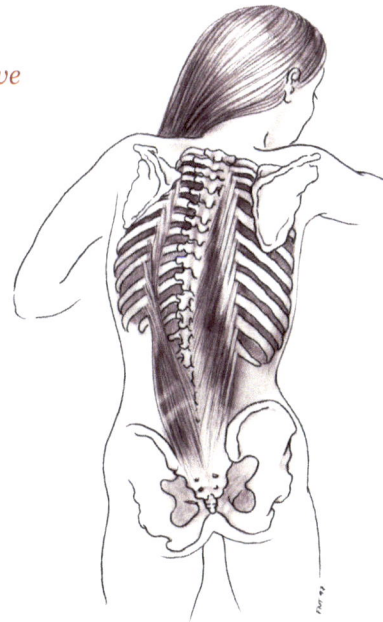

Occiput

Cervical Vertebra and Cervical Curve

Scapula

Midthoracic and
Thoracic Curve

Humerous

Lumbar Curve

Iliac Crest

Sacrum

Coccyx

Metacarpals

Femur

Tibia

Fibula

Metartarsals

Calcaneus

How your muscles are released
by doing the Side Snuzzle

The Homunculus

The homunculus is a general map
of the ratio of sensory nerves from your brain
to each part of your body.

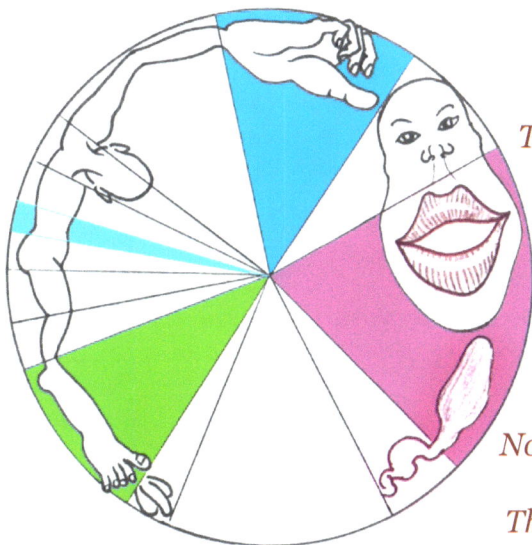

The greatest number of nerves actually is from the
area of your mouth.
The second greatest number of nerves
is to your hands;
the third most representation, i.e.,
the number of nerves,
is to your feet.

Notice the red lines showing how few sensory nerves
there are to your lower back!
This is why it is possible for you to ignore your back
pain—because you do not feel it accurately.

AN INTRODUCTION TO MOSHÉ FELDENKRAIS, D.SC.

Born in 1904, a thirteen-year old Moshé Feldenkrais journeyed alone from his home in Russia Poland to Palestine, crossing the lines of World War I. After working in Israel as a stonemason, math tutor and authoring a manual on Jiu-jitsu, Feldenkrais attended universities in Paris, France, receiving doctorates in Mechanical and Electrical Engineering and in Physics. In Paris, Dr. Feldenkrais trained with the originator of Judo, Jigaro Kano, who asked Moshé to introduce Judo to the West. Dr. Feldenkrais subsequently taught Judo and wrote *PRACTICAL UNARMED COMBAT* (1944, 1967), *JUDO: THE ART OF DEFENSE AND ATTACK* (1944, 1967), and *HIGHER JUDO* (1952).

As a physicist from 1933 to 1939, Dr. Feldenkrais assisted Joliot-Curie in the first nuclear fission research. From 1940 to 1946, Moshé designed anti-submarine warfare devices for the British Admiralty in Scotland, wrote their handbook on unarmed combat, and returned to Israel after World War II to become Director of the Electronics Department for Israel's Ministry of Defense.

It was during his work with submarines that Dr. Feldenkrais lost mobility due to an old soccer injury. Rather than undergo surgery with a poor chance of success, Moshé availed himself of the leading scientific minds in Europe in the fields of anatomy, anthropology, evolution, physiology, psychology, and infant development. Combined with his knowledge of engineering, body mechanics, and physics, Dr. Feldenkrais began to acutely observe motor development in humans and discovered the basis for his Method. His earliest books *BODY AND MATURE BEHAVIOR: A STUDY OF ANXIETY, SEX, GRAVITATION AND LEARNING* (1950) and *THE POTENT SELF* (1985) explain the scientific and psychological aspects of his work. These were followed by *AWARENESS THROUGH MOVEMENT* (1972), *THE CASE OF NORA: BODY AWARENESS AS HEALING THERAPY* (1977) and *THE ELUSIVE OBVIOUS* (1981). *THE MASTER MOVES* is an edited transcript of a workshop taught by Dr. Feldenkrais.

Moshé's insights regarding the plasticity of the newborn's nervous system and the infant's self-creation of neural pathways has only now been proven by cutting edge research, over fifty years after Moshé published his theories. Moshé was particularly pleased by his own ability to create practical applications of neurological theories and to this day he remains unparalled in his detailed perception of infant developmental movement and his translation of that movement for adults.

Even as a child Moshé had a keen awareness of how our own culture inevitably curtails each of us from achieving full neurological and emotional maturity. His own experiences of living in many cultures, and thus of seeing through many lenses, helped Moshé toward realizing his goal to transcend the cultural biases of his time. The combination of Moshé's unprejudiced vision and his skills of scientific observation were pivotal in his accurate and revolutionary perception of the workings of the human nervous system.

A highly empathetic man, Moshé carefully avoided the role of 'guru' which would have contradicted his goal that "each of you will live out your unavowed dreams" as an independent and "fully human" being. In a room filled with 300 students, Moshé was aware of the limitations, struggles, and successes of every student. He delighted in each student's success, whether it was a two-year old overcoming Cerebral Palsy, or a trainee finally discovering a movement, or a practitioner of his Method evolving in their own right. However, Moshé encouraged his students to discover their own innate ability rather than to rely on his approval and to seek being "fully human" beyond the bias and judgements of their culture. By fostering the full development of each person, Moshé deeply believed that his Method could provide a key to "a quantum leap for humanity."

ABOUT THE AUTHOR

A native of Santa Fe, New Mexico, Felicia Noelle Trujillo struggled with the crippling pain of s*pina bifida,* a birth defect of the spine. Her mother, internationally published children's artist/author Clare T. Newberry, taught her yoga from the age of five. Felicia also received massage therapy and chiropractic adjustments for six years, but her condition still left her in severe pain and repeatedly unable to walk. However, Felicia was fascinated by the world of physiotherapy and began her training in Massage Therapy and Naturopathy as a teenager and was subsequently certified in both modalities. Felicia's father, Henry V. Trujillo devoted his life to community service, first as a respected New Mexican Legislator, then as a teacher and progressive superintendent of schools.

During the 1970's, Felicia trained as a Patient Advocate at UC Medical Center/San Francisco General Hospital where she was a member of the Health Education staff and provided health education materials and medical illustration for the San Francisco County Clinical system. Until 1985, Felicia provided writing and medical illustration for physicians and four major hospitals in the Bay Area.

Felicia first met Dr. Moshé Feldenkrais in 1975, and through private sessions with him and his colleagues was able to avoid surgery for TMJ and her spine. Felicia began to realize her dream of becoming a dancer until a car accident left her with fractures of the pelvis and spine. She was informed by a neurosurgeon that she required immediate surgery, but she would still be in a wheelchair for the rest of her life.

Instead, Felicia began training with Dr. Feldenkrais and his colleagues, graduating in Israel, 1983. In 1984, Felicia continued the legacy of his work by synthesizing a new, more accessible approach to ***Feldenkrais***® movement which has kept her and her students amazingly mobile and pain free.

Moshé often encouraged the teachers he trained to develop "their own handwriting." The severity of Felicia's physical problems required that she apply ***Feldenkrais***® movement on a daily basis in order to maintain mobility. As a result, Felicia discovered a new and effective way to apply the what she calls the "neurological gestalt" of Moshé's work by synthesizing moves that only required 1-3 minutes to complete. Felicia has called this synthesis ***babymoves***™, as she primarily derived her approach from infant developmental movements and one of her innovations is teaching them in developmental sequence in her introductory course. The brilliant and insightful works of Dr. Milton Erickson and Edward T. Hall, Ph.D, have also contributed greatly to Felicia's innovative teaching.

As a teacher in international ***Feldenkrais***® Training Programs, Felicia has taught in the US, Australia, and New Zealand and has been featured in articles in all three countries. She provides Continuing Medical Education classes for medical professionals, Advanced Trainings for ***Feldenkrais***® practitioners, and popular workshops for people of all ages.

Felicia teaches a full spectrum of private students—from athletes, dancers, musicians, and martial artists to patients diagnosed with severe back pain, neuromuscular injuries, TMJ, stroke, MS, CP, Post-polio Syndrome, and CFIDS. Her specialty is teaching the "neural language" of ***babymoves***™ for the relief of the full range of back problems.

For more articles about Felicia, check her web site: *BackRescue.com*. The material presented in this *Journal* and the *Your First Moves To Rescue Your Back* series is taken from Felicia's upcoming book: ***babymoves***: **A Quantum Leap In Human Development. Please note: The *baby-moves*™ approach is not a medical or therapeutic modality, but a purely educational process.**

Great Work: A Tool Kit for Liberation

From the series Modern Day "Saints" Crafting New Realities
by Linda Braun, featured in the El Dorado Sun, June 1999

She is a tall, graceful woman, whose presence bespeaks both the wisdom of life's experiences and the openness and ease of a child.

Her father, Henry V. Trujillo, a respected legislator and teacher was introduced to her artist/author mother, Clare T. Newberry by the famous Mabel Dodge Lujan, Taos confidante of D. H. Lawrence. Unknown to their public, both her parents were part Native American.

True to the Native American and Hispanic chords in her family history, she has a long ponytail of thick, dark hair reaching to her waist. Her voice is joyous and musical as it relays a most imaginative selection of words; it's an invitation to perceive from a new seat at life's buffet table. Smiles and laughter punctuate the interaction as new possibilities arise.

Felicia Noelle Trujillo was born with the tiny imprint of a spinal defect called *spina bifida occulta.* This fact went unnnoticed and as she grew it worsened, but continued to elude diagnosis. She was in constant pain; walking was often difficult, sometimes impossible.

When Felicia was 6 years old, her mother taught her yoga, hoping it would provide relief. It didn't. Three years later, her mother discovered Jay Scherer, a Santa Fe naturopath. After a brief time as Scherer's patient Felicia told him that she wanted to do this work when she grew up. Scherer began

"I realize now how much Jay's early influence inspired me to view my work as being a form of service and spiritual practice. He also encouraged a detective approach to uncovering the source of illness; to address causes rather than symptoms."

to train her as a massage therapist and naturopath. Felicia remembers that every fall in Santa Fe meant severe asthma. She was 12 years old and weighed only 60 pounds

"I had been sitting up for 36 hours; drawing each breath was a mammoth task," she said. "My chest was like a cage, and each breath was trapped inside. My body was so painful that I suddenly felt an 'other' self that was painless and free and floated somewhere above my head looking down at myself as I sat perfectly still, laboring for the next breath.

"I woke up in the hospital, found that I could breathe more easily and fell back asleep. The next day I began to hear the screams. I rang for a nurse but no one came. It was an agonizing, pleading scream for help that continued for hours. Finally a nurse told me, 'That's just an old lady with a broken back. Her family brought her here to die 'cause she's too old to fix her back. There's nothing we can do for her.' "

"The screams woke me up again late at night. I remember my bare feet on the linoleum as I stole down the long halls, following the sound. I was frightened by just the sight of such an old woman. There were tears rolling down her wrinkled cheeks. I crept up to her side and murmured hello. Her hand shot out clutching my arm and I realized that she was blind. I was terrified. She pleaded with me in Spanish that I couldn't understand. I rang for nurses but no one came. Eventually two nurses aides passed by and I convinced them to enter the room.

" 'Oh, she just wants a bed pan,' was their translation. To my horror, the two aides yanked the old woman's legs up in the air and

forced the bed pan under her, ignoring her piercing screams. As if I were invisible, they scrabbled through the woman's things, retrieving some money and candies and left laughing. I stood there still pinned by her desperate grasp, with tears rolling down my cheeks. I swore that somehow this horrific treatment must be stopped."

Scherer, Felicia believes, had eradicated her asthma by age 14, and she returned to the very same hospital, this time as a volunteer offering massage to patients. Her struggle with the spina bifida occulta continued.

Felicia graduated from Santa Fe High in 1966 and was drawn to Northern California where Michael Murphy invited her to live at what was to become Esalen Institute. In that small, emerging community she met Alan Watts, Joan Baez, Mimi Farina, Chet Helms, Janis Joplin, Lou Gottlieb, Jack Casady, and Jerry Garcia.

In the early 1970's, hired to create the first medical graphics department for SFGH, Felicia pioneered the translation of patient information for multicultural immigrants in the Bay Area and provided health education and and medical illustration for the

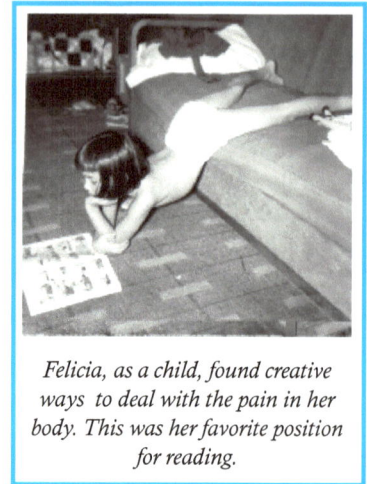
Felicia, as a child, found creative ways to deal with the pain in her body. This was her favorite position for reading.

San Francisco clinic system. As part of a team to improve health care, and drawing on her background as a naturopath, she worked to introduce innovative prenatal health education materials, breastfeeding, and assisted midwives in creating the first Alternative Birthing Center in this country. She also trained as a Patient Advocate in the UC Medical system.

One of Felicia's proudest achievements during this time came after being scrubbed and gowned to enter the nursery to do illustrations of the babies. She noticed one baby who was crying miserably and asked about his condition. The nurse replied that he was a heroin baby going through withdrawal and that nothing could be done about it.

Felicia asked if she could pick the baby up and when she did the crying stopped almost immediately. "This time," she said, "I was a grownup—and working with some of the best medical professionals in the country. They listened when I suggested we borrow a few grandmothers and granddads to come in and hold these babies. This became a national program for infants going through drug withdrawal, which I named The Cuddlers."

During these years of so much giving to others who were in pain Felicia developed severe TMJ (Temporal Mandibular Joint Dysfunction).

In 1975, friends referred her to Moshe Feldenkrais, D. Sc. His work was hands on—derived from his ability to translate evolution, neuroscience, physics, and infant development into a revolutionary approach that is said to pleasurably evoke our innate freedom of movement and true potentials on emotional, intellectual, and physical levels.

It relieved her TMJ as well as the need for surgery. And, an amazing side effect of Feldenkrais' work

was that she could walk painlessly for the first time in her life. She then proposed the notion of a hospital-based alternative clinic with the ***Feldenkrais*** Method[R] as their first innovative offering. An innovative physician, Dr. Dorothy Waddell made that into a reality.

Exuberant and able-bodied for the first time, she began to train as a dancer. Three years later a car accident left her with a fractured pelvis and the prognosis that even after surgery she would be in a wheelchair for life.

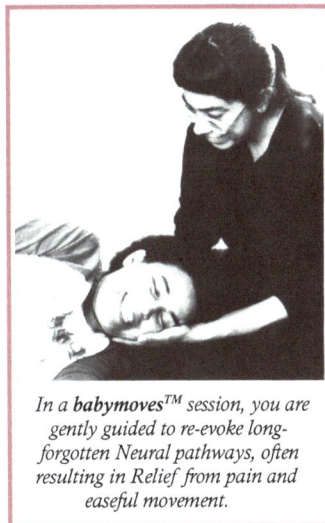

*In a **babymoves**™ session, you are gently guided to re-evoke long-forgotten Neural pathways, often resulting in Relief from pain and easeful movement.*

Once again it was the work of Moshe Feldenkrais, rather than surgery, that enabled the healing and the return of some mobility to Felicia's body. After weekly sessions she was able to walk with a cane. She received a scholarship to train with Feldenkrais in Amherst, Mass., and in his native Israel for four years, graduating in 1983. Having integrated and benefited from his work, Felicia began to synthesize her own approach which she calls ***babymoves***™.

Two years later she was free of her cane and her practice drew clients rangeing from athletes and dancers to those struggling with a variety of painful conditions.

A PERSONAL VIEW

*E**liminating pain is an enormous accomplishment; few methods are effective. Restoring or increasing the body's ability to move freely is even more astonishing. Yet this work, synthesized and created via Felicia's own life experiences, has done both for me.*

La Escuela Feliz inhabits a large adobe house with little furniture. Most of the rooms are carpeted, cosy and warm. Pillows, bolsters, and inflatable "eggs" abound, as do two wide work tables—a womblike kind of design, environment, energy. **Perfect, considering that babymoves™ unfolds from infant development and movement and merges with the evolutionary brilliance inherent in our structural design.**

I have just come through my first ***babymoves***™ session. After an initial detailed conversation about my life, Felicia has asked me to lie on the table. She uses a variety of responsive props to comfortably support my body while she works. For some of the moves I am totally passive, my body and neurology simply receiving the information supplied through these gentle movements. For some of the moves, Felicia supplies colorful, imaginative instructions to follow as I originate movements that ripple through my body. The moves themselves are delicate, rhythmic, soothing.

Lying on my back, knees bent, my left foot presses gently into the table initiating a lift in my left pelvis, which leads into a lifting of my left rib cage, then my left shoulder. Following this ripple my left arm flops over my body as I rest softly curled up on my right side. Leading with my left shoulder I return to my original position by reversing what I've just done. Felicia calls this "The Side Ripple," and I can feel it releasing spasm in my back. Much to my amazement Felicia responds with delight, "Oh, that's lovely, that's beatiful. Yes, yes, this is how you were designed to move; this is your evolutionary heritage."

Wow!, I think to myself as I melt into a full bodybeing smile, this loving acknowledgement is glorious, reawakening what must be an instinctual yearning towards full liberation.

Throughout this session I have been noticing structural changes in my body. As I lie on my back I feel my ribs relax and contact the table; my legs feel as though they extend for miles; my ribcage expands up, out and down with each breath; after my neck releases there is a new point of contact for the back of my head with the table; the angle of pelvis meeting table is different,

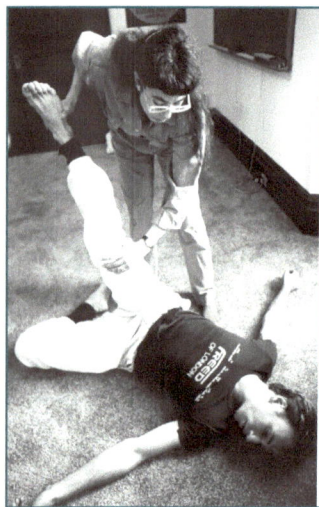

When we're finished, Felicia suggests resting (it's during rest that the body can 'file' the changes) and then moving slowly to sitting. I'm a little woozy and lightheaded; being in my body is feeling very different. Upon standing I feel and am a good bit taller than ever before. Particularly glorious is the lift and curve of

my spine and upper body. I am not making any effort, simply standing, and my spine-upper-body feels like a great sail billowed by the wind to curve gracefully upward and outward. In this case, however, it's not the wind supporting me, only my very own muscles. I was newly released from historical patterns of spasm (I was shocked to hear Felicia use the word spasm; to me they always felt 'normal'). Now my muscles were relaxed and responsive—able to be and do what they were created and designed for. A domino effect of ease and joy relays through me: from happy muscles to bones that feel newly weightless, to my vitality which feels both bouyant and grounded, to me who feels

I've suddenly been transported back to being a vivacious, playful 5-year-old.

I begin to walk around and enjoy this whoosh of energy and wildness. There's a wave of animal instinct that feels back on track. I can't help but notice that I feel very, very big and very, very free. Hmmm....feels delicious but kind of dangerous. My excitement drifts over to fear, and I start expressing my doubts to Felicia: "Isn't my chest sticking out too much? don't I look too proud, too full of myself? Somebody's not going to like this. I feel too happy, too energetic, too alive." While still strongly registering this new wave of lightness and vitality in my body, my mind is working hard to convince me that in order to preserve "myself" I'd better bail quickly.

Felicia hangs with me, gently contradicting the cultural-historical-familial mythology to which I am attempting to stay attached. What a divine place of reality, truth and comfort she holds out. I am able to disengage from my fears and tune in instead to the wisdom and perfection that my body is presenting.

Felicia comments that happy muscles feel like soft butter to the touch. When in that buttery state the "work" of "carrying" a body around ceases. Muscles are not meant to hold the body up, it's the skeleton that supports the body—your muscles get a free ride. When skeletal alignment and support happen, your body automatically becomes buoyant and light. In 'scoliosing,' the muscles are "disorganized" and pull the passive skeleton out of alighment.

Often when muscles are "holding" the body they do so in a way that goes against our true design. Here is an example: Rarely is it considered fashionable, by those who dictate those cultural commandments, to have a sway back and a derriere that sticks out. Instead, "tails" are tucked and pelvises held tight. These muscular holding patterns disrupt the natural curve of the spine that is created when a baby begins to toddle. What's more, this incorrect curve travels up the spine causing the thoracic spine and shoulders to hunch over forward. This results in pressure on the cervical spine causing, among other things, neck pain and headaches. With upper back and shoulders hunched forward, the chest is collapsed and a good deal of space designated for lungs and breathing is lost. Less oxygen is inhaled and available for use. With bones and muscles not allowed to function freely the way they were designed by a good long stretch of evolution, having a body often becomes a heavy, tense, serious experience. Odd and distressing to realize that this heavy, tense and serious body experience has become the norm for so many of us!

For most babies beginning to move and discover their bodies, all they can do is ecstatic: fingers that find their way into a mouth, toes on extended legs that swing and find fingers to clasp them. Babies revel in these simple but profound joys.

"My true goal is that you live out your unavowed dreams...." Moshe' Feldenkrais, D. Sc.

Scientific research confirms that babies create their neural pathways through these moves and interactions with their environment. This is the source of their ability to see, speak, move, rest, love and unfold as individuals.

Numerous "realities" contribute to the loss, rather than the integration, of these pleasurable, easy, moving-being experiences. By the time most people are merely a decade old they have "learned" instead to integrate a downcast perspective of disappointment, frustration, isolation and self doubt. Patterns displayed emotionally usually have their counterparts in the physical body, and vice versa.

Modern culture contributes its share of rules: Don't be too big, best to squelch your curiosity, sexuality, creativity, intelligence, etc. so that you "fit in" and "do the right thing." But even fitting in and doing the right thing does not exempt you from being typed, labeled, objectified and oppressed according to gender, sexual preference, race, religion, education and earning capacity.

What a relief to know there's a way to re-find freedom.

Felicia's work with the body, and the being that resides inside, presumes no single, right response. She trusts in the body's unique intelligence, claiming that all bodies know just what to do, but many need some guidance to get back to this original place of knowing.

What's more, Felicia's warm acceptance and encouragement of all efforts is a grand contradiction to the prevailing cultural messages that steer toward the self entrapment mentioned above.

Both she and her work present an experiential perspective that demonstrates life in a body was designed to be fun, easy, and comfortable. I share with Felicia my wonderings that if this great work were made available to everyone on

What's more, the liberation and all that follows from this is vast. Re-finding this original place of knowing coincides exactly with the wide openness of connection, compassion, respect, and love.

the planet, would peace, respect, understanding, and love flourish? She informed me that Moshe had had a similar idea. He believed that mankind was on the edge of making a quantum leap to becoming fully human. Toward that, he wanted to make his work available worldwide by broadcasting it via Sputnik.

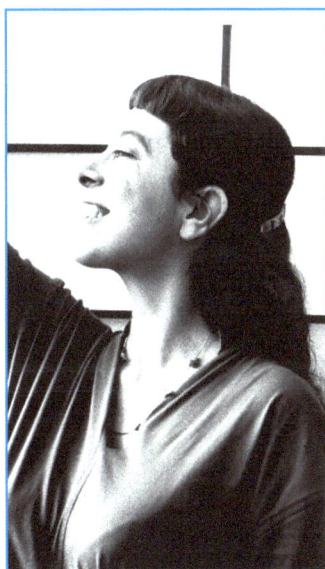

I have begun to notice, along with some of the other students at La Escuela Feliz, that in doing this work the boundaries of self and other dissolve into acceptance.

Lest you read this and think *babymoves*™ to be magic, I do want to include that working on your own is also a piece of effecting the miracle. There are a series of easy, simple moves that, when practiced regularly on your own, will continue the process of allowing your body-being to integrate this revolutionary information. As a beginner, it takes

about 30 minutes to do the moves. Felicia claims however that after doing them consistently for a year or so, you can actually do the whole series in a relaxed manner while waiting for your porridge to cook.

Felicia is particulary pleased that she was able to convince San Francisco General Hospital to include *Feldenkrai*® Practitioners in their Alternative Therapies Unit, a longtime dream of hers to allow funding and research on the efficacy of alternative treatments for the general population. They quickly earned the respect of the medical community.

"Although the 'movement lessons' are useful to anyone with a musculo-skeletal complaint which results from repetitive dysfunctional movement (runners, dancers, musicians as well as machine operators), the most dramatic benefit has been seen in individuals with severe, long-standing disability, such as paralysis due to stroke, chronic pain....or in persons with developmental handicaps.

Improvement has been seen in function as well as in relief of symptoms."

Dorothy Waddell, MD, Director Alternative Therapies Unit UC Medical Center / San Francisco General Hospital

www.backrescue.com

To experience Felicia's teaching, see BackRescue CDs & Tapes, which include journals with detailed illustrations.

RECOMMENDED BOOK LIST

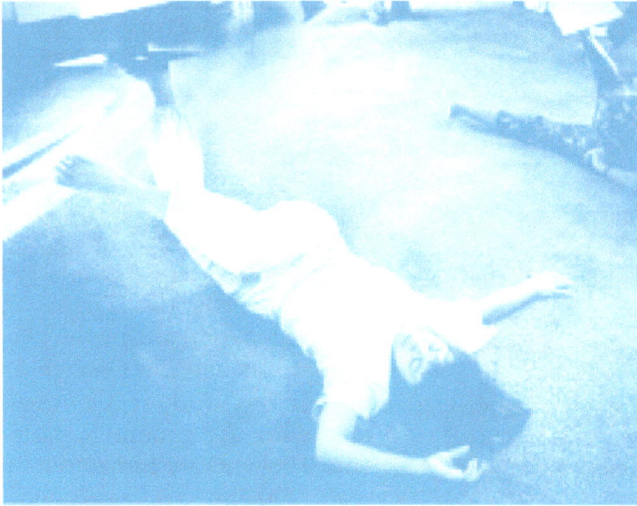

ANATOMY/NEUROPHYSIOLOGY

ANATOMY by Carmine D. Clemente;
Urban & Schwarzenberg

VOLUME 1, NERVOUS SYSTEM
by Frank Netter, MD; THE CIBA COLLECTION

THE SLIPPED DISC by James Cyriax, MD;
Charles Scribners' Sons

SURVEY OF FUNCTIONAL NEUROANATOMY
by Bill Garoutte, PhD, MD;
Jones Medical Publications

FELDENKRAIS® BOOKS

THE POTENT SELF by M. Feldenkrais, D.Sc.
BODY AND MATURE BEHAVIOR by M. Feldenkrais,
AWARENESS THROUGH MOVEMENT by M. Feldekrais
THE CASE OF NORA by M. Feldenkrais, D.Sc.
Harper & Row Publishers

MINDFUL SPONTANEITY by Ruthy Alon
Feldenkrais Resources

THE SOUNDER SLEEP SYSTEM™
Michael Krugman

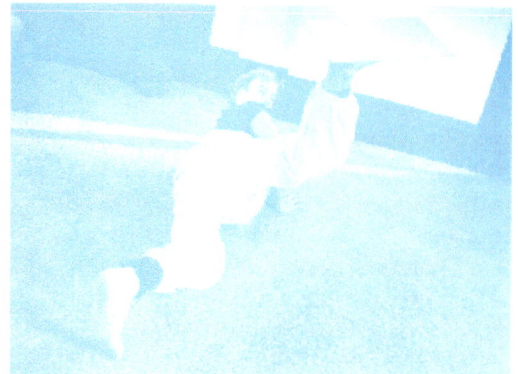

PERCEPTION/PSYCHOLOGY

UNCOMMON THERAPY: The Psychiatric
Techniques of Milton H. Erickson by
Jay Haley; W. W. Norton & Co.

THE HIDDEN DIMENSION by Edward T. Hall
THE DANCE OF LIFE by Edward T. Hall
Anchor Press/Doubleday

SCRIPTS PEOPLE LIVE by Claude Steiner
Bantam

THE CONTINUUM CONCEPT by Jean Liedhoff;
Addison-Wesley

THE UNFASHIONABLE HUMAN BODY
by Bernard Rudofsky (sadly, out of print)

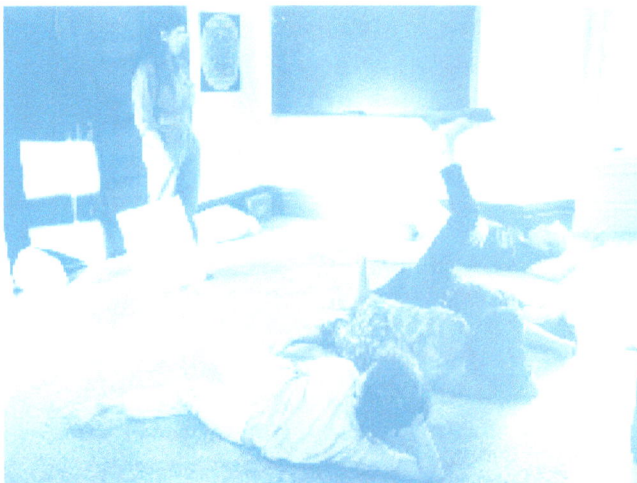

www.ingramcontent.com/pod-product-compliance
Lightning Source LLC
Chambersburg PA
CBHW060825270326
41931CB00002B/70